LOVE YOUR NEW SKINNY

A guide to finding the right exercise program that fits your life without having to give up what makes you happy

Cressida Thomas

DISCLAIMER

Cressida Thomas

This book is dedicated to Jamie, Cassie, and Joshua who have my heart always.

It is also dedicated to everyone who has searched for a fitness plan that is filled with joy and adventure. May you find it and fill it with joy and abundance.

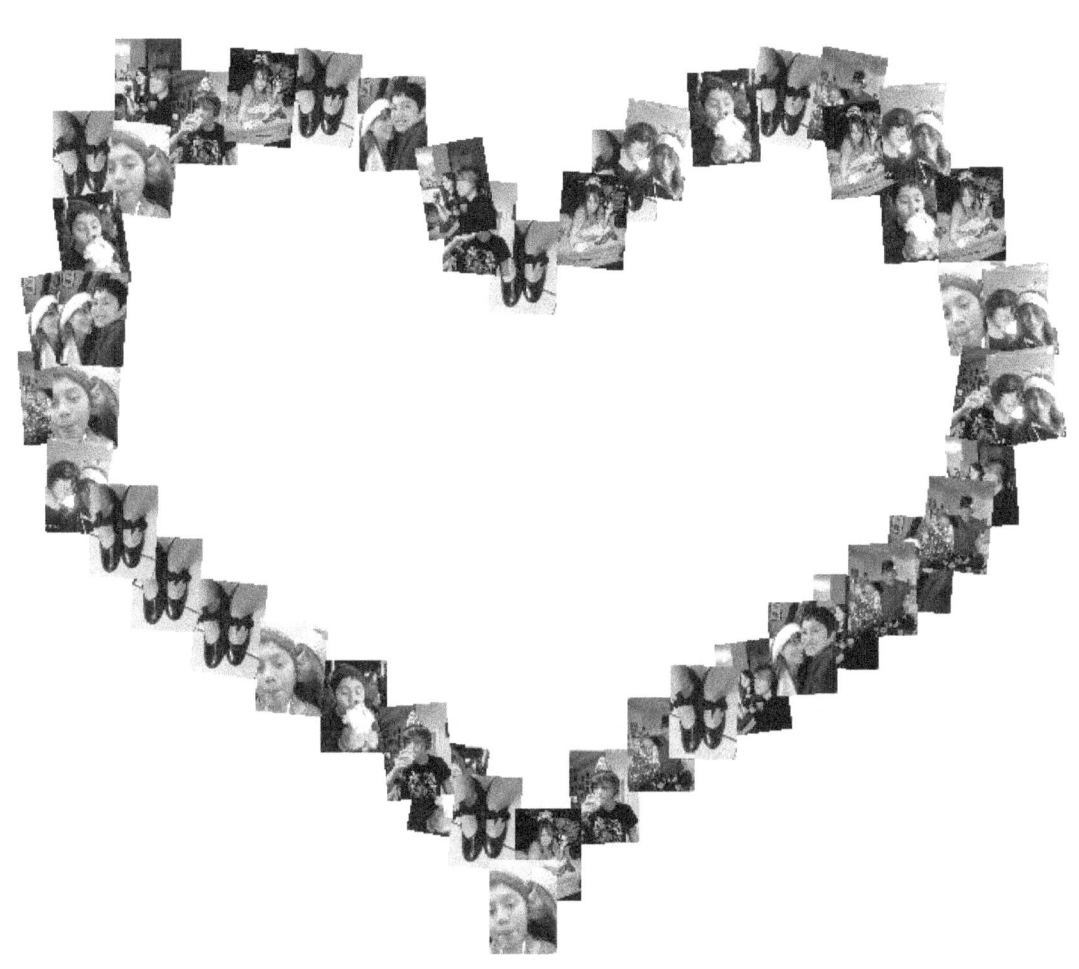

Table of Contents

Love Your New Skinny

Introduction

Here is my own fitness plan for "my skinny". It is a plan that helps me maintain my weight, while still eating the things I like. For years I tried new diets and fitness plans, only to slowly give up, while gaining my weight back. Why didn't I stick with these plans? One, I wasn't having any fun. Two, the fitness plans were either too time consuming or too much money. Sound familiar? If so, I have a better plan for you. At age forty-four(yes I've said it) and three teen agers later I have pieced together a plan for healthy living that works for me. I do not feel deprived. I can eat what I want. I can fit into my jeans. And most importantly I HAVE FUN AND FEEL GOOD ABOUT MYSELF! You can use my plan altogether, or take the pieces that work for you and make it your own. I have found a fitness plan is like a quilt. I take the most loved pieces, make them work together, and wrap myself around it.

I don't believe exercise or dieting should hurt. I should never feel injured or deprived. Those types of feelings imbeds in my brain and do not keep me coming back. This is why many fitness plans do not work for me. They take away things I enjoy and replace them with things I do not. No one can tell me how to exercise. Only I know which types I enjoy and will look forward to each day.

Don't listen to what others tell you to do. Listen to your body. What works for one person doesn't necessarily work for you and so forth.

Many of my friends fit in gym time in the morning. I have three teen agers to get out the door and do not have time for a morning work- out. I do, however, manage to stretch, meditate, and greet each morning(rather quickly) before I dash out the door. Whatever time works for you **use** it. There are no *wrong* ways. If I do go to the gym, I prefer the company of my son. I pick a time soon after dinner, when things are quieter at home, to go over to the gym and swim with my son. I do not rush. I don't see the point in rushing something I enjoy. The benefits are bounteous. I spend quality time with my son and stay fit at the same time.

Many people have home gyms as well. I have a small one I created with little money. You would be surprised at how easy this is to do. Your "gym" doesn't have to be fancy to be efficient.   Some items in my gym are as follows:

1. Yoga mat
2. Free Weights
3. A Kettle Bell

4. Ballet Shoes

5. Tap Shoes

6. A Small Gym Bike

7. Boxing Gloves

8. A small peddler exercise bike

9. A small set of a variety of workout dvds

This may seem like a lot but don't get discouraged. I acquired these items over a long period of discovering what I **enjoy doing**. I tried different things out. Kept what I liked and gave away what I didn't. You can create your own **gym**. Be creative and challenge yourself. Make it fun and make it your own!

On a side note, I was given advice from a friend who I think of as my "gym master." I was told to **STAY OFF THE SCALE**. I know this is a scary idea. It feels a little out of control. The reason I for stay off the scale is there are so many factors in determining my daily weight. I get discouraged if my weight fluctuates. My friend explained to me if that if I feel good and can wear the clothes I love then I am at the correct weight. This is not in any way professional advice. It is, however, advice that makes sense to me. If I can fit into my favorite clothes and like how I feel and look, then I am at the correct weight. **End of scale story.**

Take time to read through this book. Write down any ideas that come to you. Have fun in creating your own fitness plan and love your new skinny!

Find Your New Skinny

What is your "new skinny"? Put simply, it's the weight you feel *healthy* with. It's the one when   you can fit into your favorite pair of jeans and say "HELLO WORLD. THIS IS ME". Walk out that door. Smile and strut.   For everyone, this goal may look different because we were *all made* to look different. It's how we *feel* that is most important. The voyage we take to reach our fitness goals are unique.   How do we reach our goals? Break out your notebook and get ready for your "new skinny"!

Chapter One:

Your New Skinny Rules:

1. **"Think Skinny" attitude.** Think "Skinny" and center yourself: I realize this is a confusing concept so let me break it down to you in simple terms. Do not think of yourself as "not skinny". I believe in the law of attraction. If I think *fat* I will probably *feel* fat. I won't lose much weight with these negative thoughts. Choose to think *skinny thoughts*. Let me explain how this works for me. First, I create a visual of ideas that remind me of staying fit. I have found that visual charts are very powerful tools for me. I can bring about just about anything I **look** at enough. I can look at pictures of yoga and I feel energized and motivated. This is how powerful and image can be. I also enjoy making these charts because they are fun to do. There are many ways to make them and the best part of this is you can choose any way you would like. The way I choose to make my "Skinny Chart Visual" is by making a chart on my computer. You can make yours using paper and cut out magazine pictures. You can also make it by

simply drawing what being fit and skinny looks like to you. Whichever way works for you is great. Just make sure it is not costly and can be accessed frequently throughout the day. My "Skinny chart" visual is free. I just use free pictures on the internet and clip and paste them to an open document on my computer. I keep my laptop close to me and my tablet even closer! I have a program on my tablet that opens my Skinny Chart instantly. I then look at all of the fun pictures I have pasted and I raise my level of consciousness to a "place of fit". I'm ready to face the day new. The visual chart you will make needs to be filled with positive visuals of how you would like to see yourself. My chart is filled with endless pictures of the ways I see myself feeling fit and skinny. For example, I happen to love yoga. I have many fun pictures of what yoga means to me. It motivates me to feel calm and ready to start my yoga routine. I also have pictures of weights. I enjoy weight lifting and this motivates me to want to lift weights. I throw in other pictures as well, such as new outfits I plan to wear and hair styles. This helps complete the picture of how I want to see myself. Smiling, doing yoga with a new scarf in my hair! I look at my skinny chart though out the day. It is a very powerful tool. If possible, choose a program to make your chart that can be downloaded to your smart phone if you have one. I can access my skinny chart wherever I am. I do this at the market, in the parking lot of my children's school, and in my bed before I go to sleep. The results are fabulous. I do more yoga, lift weights, and I now wear scarves in my hair! What I create on my skinny board happens! This is one of the tools I use to become the fit and skinny me I am. Make your chart your own and own it!

Chapter Two

2. **The New Skinny "ATTACK FOODS"**

I specifically like this section because we get to talk about FOOD! I love food. Most people do. I just don't like a. gaining weight and b. feeling bloated. So I have constructed a list of yummy foods I call "attack foods". They are the ones that taste great, fill me up, and more importantly, they are not high in fat and help me to be healthy. In other words they "attack" the craving to grab an unhealthy snack. Most diets tell you what to eat which I find ridiculous. Personally, I cannot eat many things other people can. I believe everyone's body is absolutely different from one another. What digests easily in your body many not digest well in mine . I also like different things than you do. I cannot eat what so many diets tell me to because the foods may cause me to feel sick. I also may not even *like* the foods they suggest. For example, I cannot and will not eat unnatural cheese. Cheese that has been chemically altered to be "fat free" and do not melt in the microwave is not "food" to me. These cheeses taste like clay and give me a stomach ache. That being said, I choose naturally low-fat cheeses, such as provolone. It's a great tasting, naturally low-fat cheese that brings me pleasure without the fat. If you have not caught on yet I LOVE CHEESE. To eliminate cheese from my life would not make me happy and my goal is to stay happy and healthy. I do not deprive myself of cheese. I do, however, stay conscious of the amount of cheese I need in my food to be healthy and feel satisfied. To my surprise it doesn't take much. I can add an ounce or two of my favorite shredded cheese to a plate full of lettuce and wah lah! It not only tastes great but is naturally low fat. I get to eat cheese and stay thin.

So now let's get on with my list of Skinny Mom Attack Foods:

Shredded Cheese: Your favorite cheese can be shredded or even cut in pieces but it's important that it is portioned out. I can eat cheese on anything but it's the amount that keeps me healthy. I do not need to have a cup of cheese to feel happy, in fact, if I eat too much cheese I don't even feel good. So my first attack food is having a bag of shredded cheddar cheese available in my fridge to "toss" onto anything I please. I try to eyeball an ounce. If you need to weigh it do so. After a while you will know by site what an ounce is. Remember, an ounce of cheese goes a long way you will see!

Frozen Steak Fries: Another favorite here! I love fries. Frozen "steak" fries that are oven baked are low in fat and delicious. They are also easy to season and are satisfyingly filling.   Bake them golden brown and you can add pepper for taste. Steak sauce is a low-fat condiment and is delicious with fries. Want to add zest? Add hot sauce to them! There are so many low fat ideas for oven baked fries and zero guilt in eating them.

Lettuce: For those of you who love salad, buying the pre-prepared salads are an easy way to instantly add love to your plate. I rarely go a meal without any lettuce. If you want to save money, buy lettuce and prepare it ahead of time so you can throw it into any meal. Lettuce goes with everything! Throw a bulk of lettuce onto your plate, an ounce of shredded cheese, toss it around with vinegar(a tasty zero fat dressing) and top it off with salsa and you have a mouthful of goodness. Want some sweet with your zest? Cut up some banana and throw it on! Add an ounce of chicken or beef and make it a taco salad! It's that easy. It's filling and delicious. You don't have to deprive yourself of flavor. Just be bulk up on the green and be mindful of the rest!

The Fruit and Veggie Zone: We all know that anything green and that is a fruit is a great addition to our plate. Personally, I have to be careful of which fruits and veggies I choose because not all digest the same. Choose which ones are right for you and keep them on hand. **Bananas** are a personal favorite for me. They satisfy my sweet tooth and fill me up, leaving me with lots of brain power. A bowl of carrots and mushrooms are delicious with hot sauce sprinkled on top. I never have to go "dip free" again if I choose the right dips. I try to "bulk" my meals up with green beans seasoned with pepper and have even had an artichoke as a main dish. Prepared without fat, vegetables and fruits are always a great food investment and tastes great too!

Soda Crackers This may seem strange but soda crackers are naturally lower in fat than chips and taste great with salsa. I eat them when I need a quick snack pick up. They also go great along with a green salad topped with salsa.

Salsa!! I cannot say enough about a great salsa. Salsa is a naturally low fat food and tastes great with just about anything. It can be used as a dip or even a salad dressing. I can prepare my own, or buy it, either way it adds love to everything I eat.

This is a list of some of my "**attack foods**". They are all easy to buy and prepare in a way that you like. Just make sure what you add with it is healthy too. Be creative. Find foods and make them your own ATTACK FOODS!

Chapter Three

EXERCISE YOUR WAY

Exercise has unlimited power. It helps you burn calories and also makes you feel good. By exercising, we can actually sends messages to our brains that make us happy. So why does it feel like a chore to many people? Putting it simply: Many people find exercises that are **painful** and **boring**. The people that say "no pain, no gain, are just trying to convince you to do it "their way". Their way may work for them but it may not for you. I am not saying that I don't feel sore at times when exercise. Usually when I'm having fun kickboxing I am not aware of any pain. I'm too busy having fun which is the point. **Have fun**. Now afterward, I may be a bit sore. But it's a *good* sore because I know I had fun and will do it again tomorrow. The way that I have been able to maintain my "exercise life" is by doing things that **1. I have fun doing 2. Do not cause a lot of pain**. Unfortunately, we all have to try some things we may not like to find what we *do like*. I had to experiment a lot to find the kinds of exercises I like that keep me coming back for more. The fun part in this discovery is the voyage. Find types of exercises that excite you. I tried a variety of inexpensive exercise dvds to find out which ones I liked. It was a small investment and the great part is I now can switch back and forth from one exercise to another depending on my mood. One day I may box, another day I may do belly dancing. **Get creative**. Try things you never thought you could do.   Two years ago I began to try out a ballet workout tape. I fumbled around copying what the instructor was telling me, while feeling glamorous in the comfort of my room. I probably did not look so graceful but that part doesn't matter. I felt glamorous and therefore, I was **glamorous.**   See how that works? And guess what I do now? I now attend a local ballet school with my two daughters and get to feel pretty special in a real dance room. I started with an idea, baby stepped to an exercise video, then dove into a real life experience.   After trying ballet I began tap dance.   I now get to feel like Ginger Rogers once a week. First a dream... **Now reality**. I also get the benefit of yes...staying fit!   Place these types of dreams into your "Skinny board" and watch them manifest.   Remember you can take baby steps or dive in all at once. You have nothing to lose...but the extra weight!

More about exercise...not everyone wants to use exercise videos for working out. There are plenty of enjoyable ways to exercise without them. You can make your routine as simple or complicated as you like. You may want to take a walk each day or even go for a jog in a local park. The opportunities are endless and do not have to cost anything. Some people really love going to the gym. Some people would rather play a dance game on their gaming system. The opportunities for exercise are endless. The ones you choose should be fun. One day I may choose to do yoga and another day I may meet a friend at the gym. Recently I played Wi Ski on our video game system. I went skiing in my living room. 80 calories burned. Some days I put on my belly dance skirt and practice in my living room. Burn calories and have fun. It's a win/win.

Be creative. I have coached my son's baseball team and found this is a great way to exercise. I not only burned calories but had fun, added to the community, and created memories with my son. How better than that can it get? The possibilities for exercise are endless. Open yourself up to new ideas and dive in.

On a quick note..I'd like to thank Virginia Hey, actress(Mad Max, Farscape) for introducing me to the world of Zumba Dance. **She told me I could do it and I did.** She is a strong, beautiful woman and a great inspiration to me.

Chapter Four

Meditate the "New Skinny" way: I cannot say enough about meditation. It helps me stay calm and centers me. I include this in my fitness program because when I am centered I make good choices which include food and exercise ones. I maximize my meditations with yoga. There are many different kinds of yoga and many videos and books written on this subject. I have tried a bit of them all and each one teaches me to stay **centered** and be **present**. Being present is key to exercise and eating well. What do I mean by being present? It means I am quieting my mind and focusing on what I am doing right **now**. I make my plate of food and I say a prayer of **gratitude** for it. I eat slowly. I chew each bite and wash it down with water. Water is the only drink I will have with meals. I can easily forget to drink enough and become dehydrated. Water really is essential to my health. I have learned that many times when I think I am hungry what I really am is "**thirsty**". I drink water throughout the day. I drink it while exercising and with every meal. I take it on the go and keep it with me at all times. Mediation can come in all forms. While eating I like to slow down into a meditative type state. I taste all of my bites. The food goes down more easily and digests properly. I don't rush any meals. I drink plenty of water while eating. The longer I take to eat the better able my body is to tell me when I am **full** and nourished. My body knows what it wants and needs. I just have to slow down to hear it.

More about meditation. Again, finding your own meditation method may take time. Do some research on which methods work for you. Remember to keep it simple. Choose a way to mediate that is enjoyable. Remember if it isn't fun you may not stick with it. **Breathing is key to meditation**. Take many moments throughout the day to breathe slower. **Observe your surroundings**. The more joy I find in my world the better I eat, the more I want to exercise and listen to my body. All of these things are connected. **Listen to your inner self.** Let your body tell you what you need. Listen to crickets, rain, birds, whichever sounds that put you in your joyful space. I often do yoga stretches, along with my meditations. I burn calories while finding "**my inner happy place**".

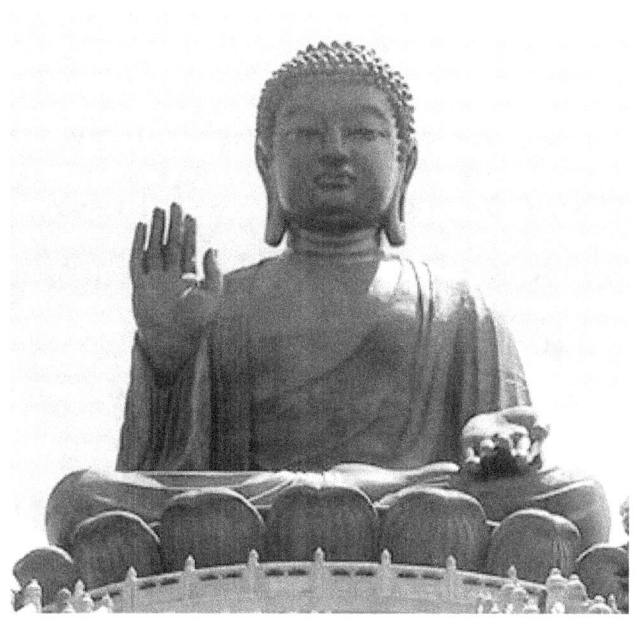

Chapter Five

All the rest…..The ideas I've presented so far are all tools I've personally incorporated in my life to achieve and maintain my weight and more balanced lifestyle. All of my tools are simple because I can't maintain anything that is more complicated. There are other notes I'd like to share that aren't in a category of their own but are important to my weight management.

I get plenty of rest. This is simple to write and not always easy to do. I have a rule not to do anything stressful two hours before I go to bed. This includes talking to my family or friends about any stressful matter if I don't have to. There are circumstances when I do have to talk about important matters, however, these are the exceptions to the rule. I give myself an hour or two of winding down time. I may read a book or watch a comedy but everyone has a different way to center themselves before bed. If I can even manage ten minutes of yoga and meditation my sleep is better. I go to bed at the same time each night(I may stretch it a little on the week-ends but not by much) and I usually get up at the same time each morning The times may be different for each person but the concept is the same. Give yourself some quiet down time before bed. Have a regular routine and get the hours of sleep you need to feel good. This leads to good daily food choices and the ability to plan out your exercise time.

I am "present" for my family and friends. What I mean by "present" is I take time to give my full attention to my kids and a few friends each day. I am a realist. My day is full like everyone else and it's often tricky to be fully present to everyone all of the time. I try to "check in" with my kids each day beyond the regular daily routine. I also try to do this with some of my closest friends. By doing this, I make a big investment in my "**joy jar**". All of my best moments go there. How does filling my jar of joy contribute to my health? A full joy jar leads to a happy and more relaxed me. This leads to more good food and exercise choices.

What is your **new skinny**? It's the best and most healthy **you.** It is the you that follows a living plan full of yummy healthy food choices that **you like**. It's the you that takes time to do an exercise that **you enjoy**. I have incorporated these ideas into my daily living and by doing so I have the ability to be the best skinny me possible. We live in a world that consistently gives us unhealthy body images. Take your power back and choose how you **eat, exercise**, and **see yourself**. Choose to be **happy** and **healthy. Choose to love your new skinny!**

Chapter Six

How It All Comes Together….

It fascinates me how every aspect of my life attributes to weight management and good health. In writing what my weight loss/maintenance plan is I hope that I have kept it simple enough to understand, yet roomy enough for you to "make it your own." A positive attitude is a great beginning. Open yourself up to all exercise opportunities.   Make a visual "skinny chart" and use it to manifest how you want to look and feel. Be **creative** and practice **faith**. Know that your goals will happen.

Have on hand the "**attack foods**" I listed that work for you and create some of your own. Share your ideas!

Make exercise your own personal adventure. Find what makes you happy and endeavor at things you've dreamed about.

Take time to **meditate** and incorporate this into your exercise. You'd be surprised at how many calories can be burned by sitting still.

Make time to feel joy in your life. Joy leads to a life filled with love. Healthy choices naturally follow………..

Frequently Asked Questions

1. How do I find time to meditate in my busy schedule?

Most everyone is busy and finding a time and place to meditate can be challenging. The time and place you do your meditation is not as important as long as you do make time. I have found myself meditating after dropping my kids off at school. I have taken time to meditate in the bathroom while washing my face. Your time could even be while you eat your breakfast or have your first cup of coffee. As long as you remember to breathe slowly and think positive thoughts any time can be "meditation time".

2. How do I find time to exercise?

As I state in my book, there are many opportunities to exercise. Not everyone's schedule is the same. Look at each day and decide when you can fit in small increments of exercise. I have found that while watching a movie with my kids I can use my free weights. This also keeps me from turning to the "munchies" and is fun.

3. Where do I start?

Start off by reading this book and writing your notes for your own fitness plan. Create your own "skinny chart" visual. Make a plan to try one new form of exercise that excites you. Start out slowly and enjoy the process.

4. What do you do during football season?(I threw this question in myself!)

I wanted to include this question because the topic can be applied to any event. I love football. I also love the snacks associated with football. I love chicken wings, chips, and yes..salsa! During a game day or any other special occasion I can still apply all of my personal rules. I can choose to eat two delicious wings. I can eat them slowly and happily. I can choose to eat fewer tortilla chips than I do bagel chips and make sure I fill them with salsa. I can go for a walk during half time. These ideas, while simple, can be easily applied to any occasion.

I hope that you find my tools work for you as they work for me. I wish you joy, happiness, and health....
Namaste,

Cressida

About the author...

Cressida Thomas is a writer and a proud mother of three teenagers. She currently attends Hartnell College and resides in Salinas, California. Cressida is a member of Phi Theta Kappa Honor Society and a three-time graduate of the Salinas Adult School Pre-School Co-op program. Her experience includes work at Lucille Packard Children's Hospital at Stanford and has written for nutrition publications for W.I.C.

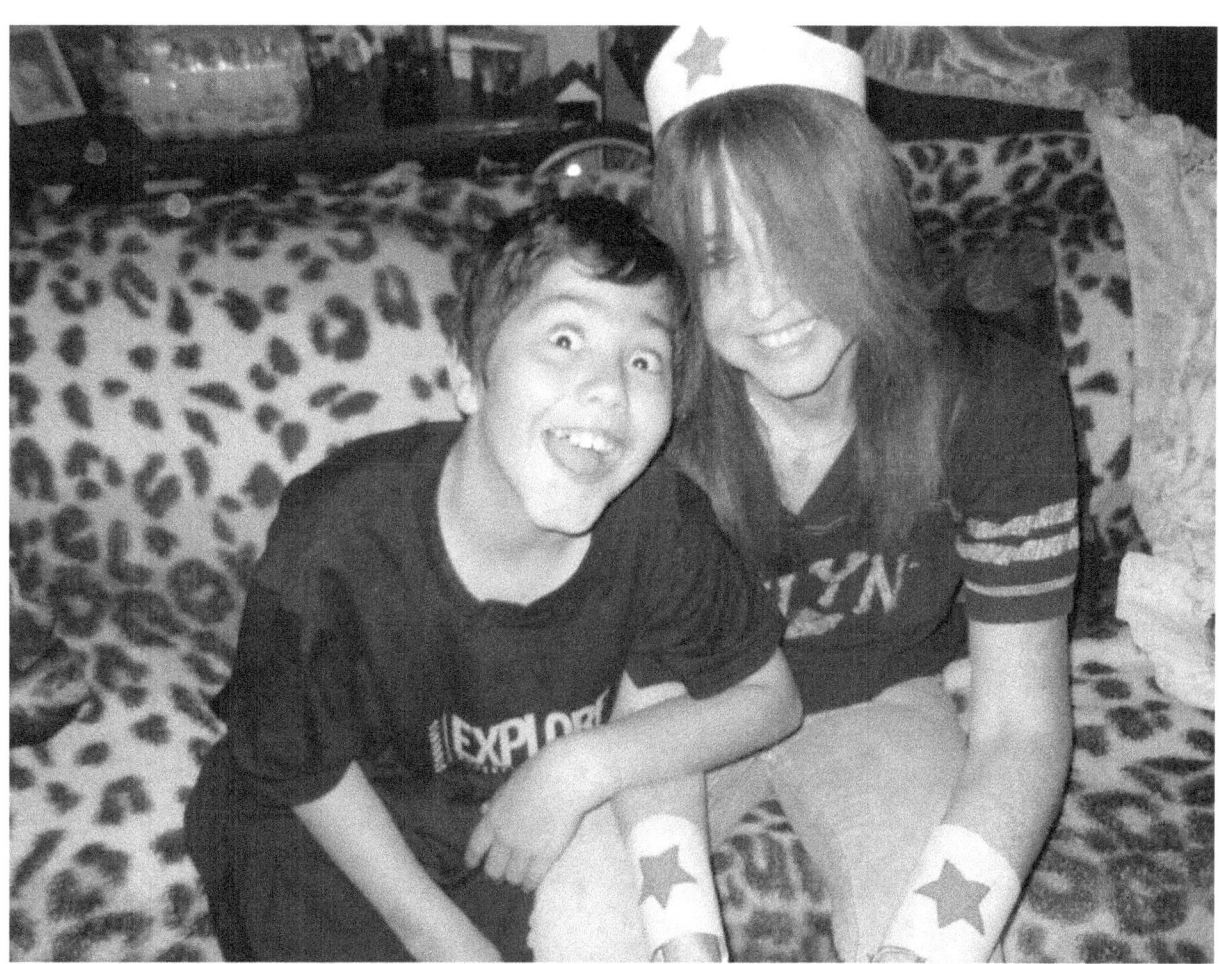

Other Books by Cressida Thomas

The Three Love Principles (also available on Kindle)

Before you go...if you are reading this on your kindle will you take a moment to share your thoughts?

Thank you and many blessings....